I0421480

The Paleo Guide Book

Including Food Lists and 25 Delicious Recipes

Disclaimer and Terms of Use:

Effort has been made to ensure that the information in this book is accurate and complete, however, the author and the publisher do not warrant the accuracy of the information, text and graphics contained within the book due to the rapidly changing nature of science, research, known and unknown facts and internet. The Author and the publisher do not hold any responsibility for errors, omissions or contrary interpretation of the subject matter herein. This book is presented solely for motivational and informational purposes only.

Table of Contents

Introduction 5

About the Paleo Diet 7

Paleo Diet Recipes..................................... 10

    Tomato Basil Omelet 12

    Banana Coconut Flour Pancakes 14

    Strawberry, Spinach and Banana Smoothie......... 16

    Sautéed Sweet Potato Hash 18

    Almond Flour Blueberry Muffins 20

    Triple Berry Coconut Smoothie 22

    Cinnamon Spiced Pumpkin Pancakes 24

    Raspberry Coconut Muffins 26

    Cream of Broccoli Soup..................... 28

    Spinach Salad with Strawberries 30

    Dairy-Free Chicken Pecan Salad 32

    Creamy Carrot Ginger Soup 34

    Spring Salad with Mango, Avocado and Walnuts. 36

    Egg Salad with Fresh Chives 38

    Coconut-Crusted Baked Haddock 40

    Rosemary Roasted Chicken..................... 42

    Herb-Roasted Pork Tenderloin 44

    Bacon-Wrapped Scallops 46

Easy Homemade Meatloaf 48

Spicy Chipotle Turkey Burgers 50

Cinnamon Baked Bananas 52

Chocolate Fudge Brownies 53

Coconut Vanilla Cupcakes 55

Blueberry Almond Flour Crisp 57

Avocado Chocolate Mousse 59

Conclusion 61

Introduction

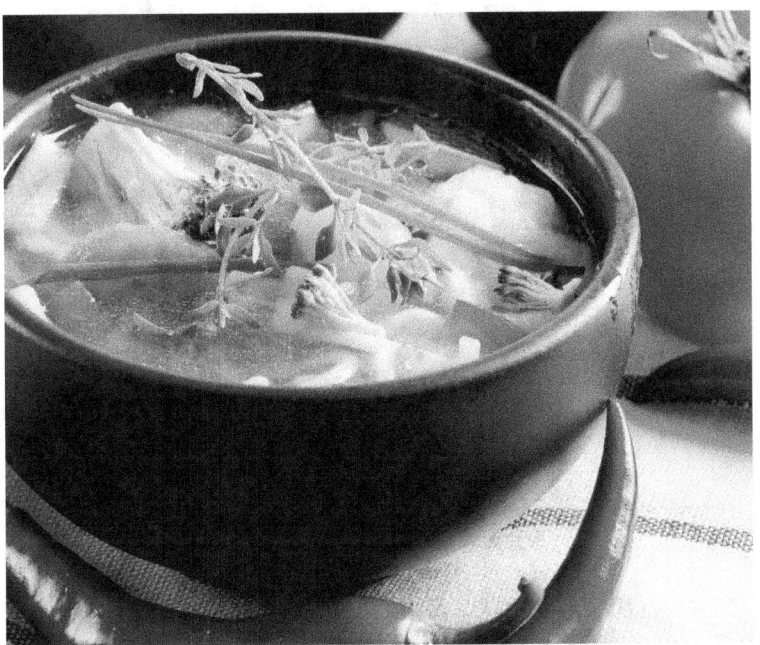

The Paleo Diet is based on the dietary habits of our Paleolithic-era ancestors and it is rapidly gaining popularity. In addition to being a great tool for weight loss, the Paleo Diet may help to relieve the symptoms of a variety of serious health problems including diabetes, heart disease, and more. In this book you will receive an introduction to the Paleo Diet including lists of foods to eat and avoid as well as some key information about the diet. By the time you finish this book you will have the knowledge you need to get started with the Paleo Diet – you will also receive a collection of twenty-five delicious Paleo recipes including breakfast, lunch, dinner, and dessert options.

About the Paleo Diet

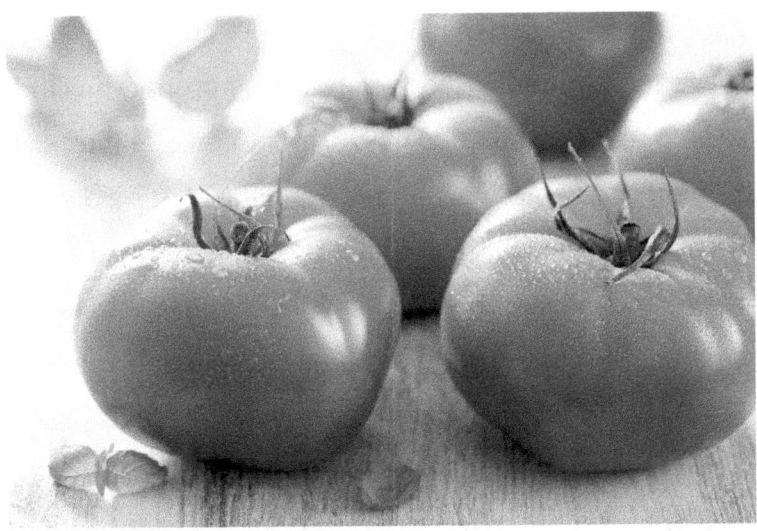

As you may already know, the Paleo diet is based around the eating habits of our Paleolithic-era ancestors. During the Paleolithic era, humans lived hunter-gatherer lifestyles – they did not plant crops or keep livestock, they simply lived off the land. The Paleo diet includes those foods which would have been available to humans at that time as well as other foods that do not require processing or refinement to make them safe for human consumption. Products of agriculture like dairy products, grains, and legumes are not included in the Paleo diet – neither are sugars, artificial sweeteners, processed foods, fast foods, and many snack foods.

The Paleo diet is founded on the principles of whole food nutrition – foods should be prepared with as little alteration as possible. The benefits of the Paleo diet are many. Not only does this diet help you to improve your nutrition and therefore your overall health and wellbeing, but it may also help you to lose weight, to improve the symptoms of chronic diseases like diabetes and heart disease, and to improve your energy levels and concentration. While it may be challenging to get used to the restrictions of the diet at first, the Paleo diet is really quite simple.

Below you will find a general list of the foods you should be eating on the Paleo diet:

- Fresh fruits, including dried fruit
- Fresh vegetables and herbs
- Eggs and lean protein
- Fresh fish and seafood
- Nuts and seeds (except peanuts)
- Avocado, olives and olive oil
- Grain-free, gluten-free flours
- Coffee, herbal tea and fruit juice

Switching to a new diet can be confusing but if you are serious about improving your health, losing weight, or simply changing your lifestyle, then the Paleo diet is an excellent tool. The Paleo diet is not complicated and you do not have to count calories if you do not want to. Simply remove grains, dairy, and sugar from your diet in favor of fresh fruits and vegetables, nuts and seeds, healthy fats and oils, eggs, seafood, and lean protein. If you are ready to give the Paleo diet a try, simply pick a recipe from this book and get started!

Paleo Diet Recipes

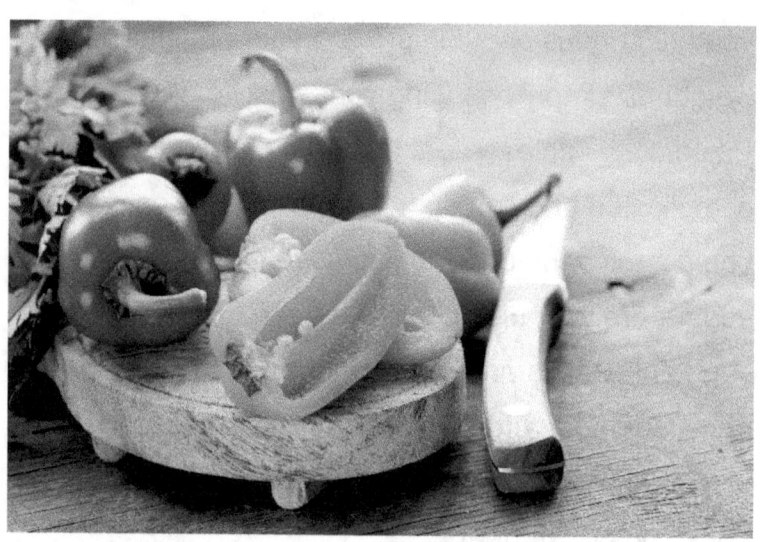

Recipes Included in this Book:

Tomato Basil Omelet

Banana Coconut Flour Pancakes

Strawberry, Spinach, Banana Smoothie

Sautéed Sweet Potato Hash

Almond Flour Blueberry Muffins

Triple Berry Coconut Smoothie

Cinnamon Spiced Banana Pancakes

Raspberry Coconut Muffins

Cream of Broccoli Soup

Spinach Salad with Strawberries

Dairy-Free Chicken
Pecan Salad

Creamy Carrot Ginger
Soup

Spring Salad with Mango,
Avocado Walnut

Egg Salad with Fresh
Chives

Coconut-Crusted Baked
Haddock

Rosemary Roasted
Chicken

Herb-Roasted Pork
Tenderloin

Bacon-Wrapped Scallops

Easy Homemade
Meatloaf

Spicy Chipotle Turkey
Burgers

Cinnamon Baked
Bananas

Chocolate Fudge
Brownies

Coconut Vanilla
Cupcakes

Blueberry Almond Flour
Crisp

Avocado Chocolate
Mousse

Tomato Basil Omelet

Servings: 1

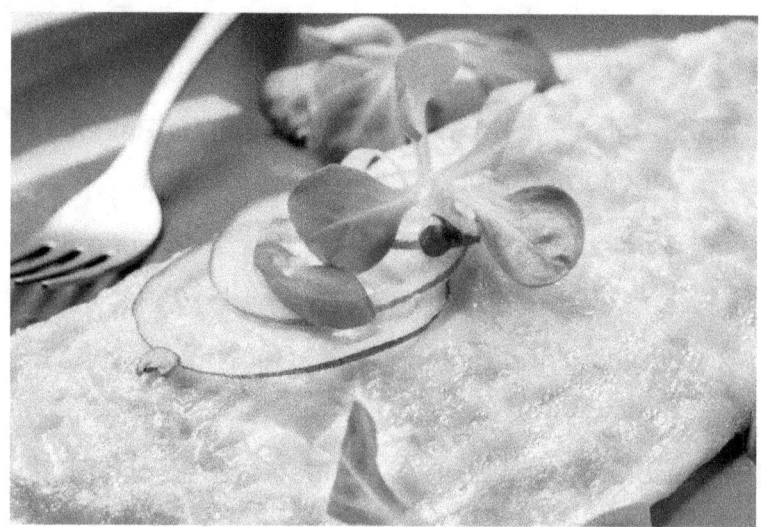

Ingredients:

2 teaspoons olive oil, divided

1 medium ripe tomato, chopped

2 tablespoons diced yellow onion

1 clove garlic, minced

2 large eggs

1 tablespoon chopped chives

Salt and pepper to taste

Instructions:

1. Heat 1 teaspoon of oil in a small skillet over medium heat.
2. Add the tomato, onion, and garlic – cook for 3 to 4 minutes until tender.
3. Spoon the vegetables off into a bowl then reheat the skillet with the remaining oil.
4. Whisk together the egg, chives, salt and pepper then pour into the skillet.
5. Cook for 2 minutes or until the egg is almost set.
6. Spoon the vegetables over half the omelet and sprinkle with basil.
7. Fold the empty half of the omelet over the filling and cook for another minute or until the egg is set.

Banana Coconut Flour Pancakes

Servings: 4

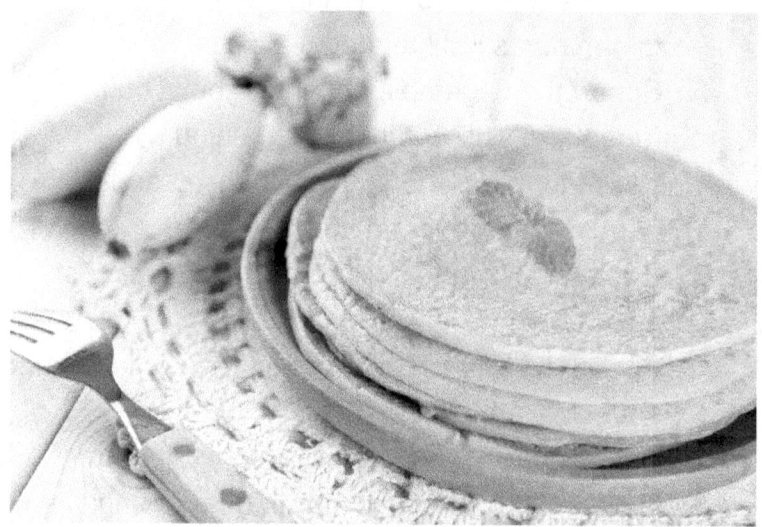

Ingredients:

4 medium ripe bananas, peeled and sliced

6 large eggs, whisked

¼ cup plus 2 tablespoons coconut flour

½ teaspoon ground cinnamon

Pinch salt

Instructions:

1. Combine the bananas, coconut flour, eggs, cinnamon and salt in a food processor.
2. Blend until smooth and well combined.

3. Heat a skillet over medium-high heat and grease with cooking oil.
4. Spoon the batter into the pan, using about 2 to 3 tablespoons per pancake.
5. Cook for 1 to 2 minutes until the underside is lightly browned.
6. Flip the pancakes and cook for another 2 minutes or until browned on the underside.
7. Transfer the pancakes to a plate to keep warm and repeat with the remaining batter.

Strawberry, Spinach and Banana Smoothie

Servings: 1 to 2

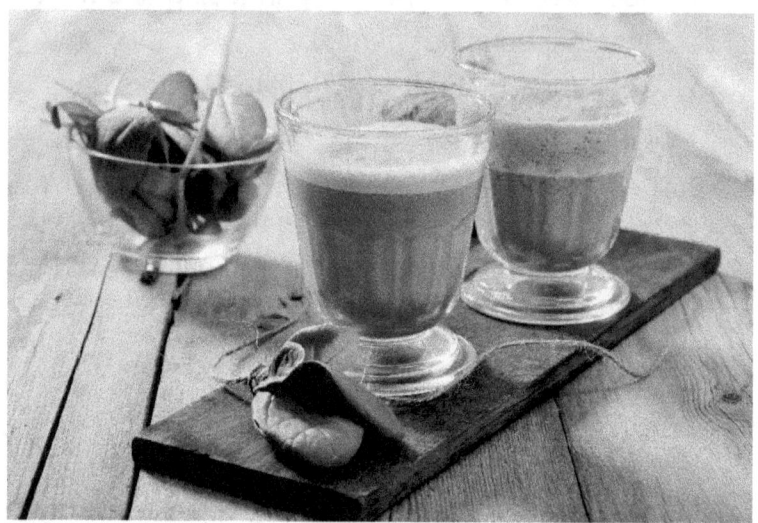

Ingredients:

2 cups fresh chopped spinach

1 cup frozen sliced strawberries

1 medium frozen banana, peeled and sliced

1 cup unsweetened almond milk

½ cup ice cubes

1 tablespoon raw honey

Instructions:

1. Combine all of the ingredients in a high-speed blender.

2. Blend for 30 to 60 seconds until smooth and well combined.
3. Divide the smoothie among two glasses and serve immediately.

Sautéed Sweet Potato Hash

Servings: 4

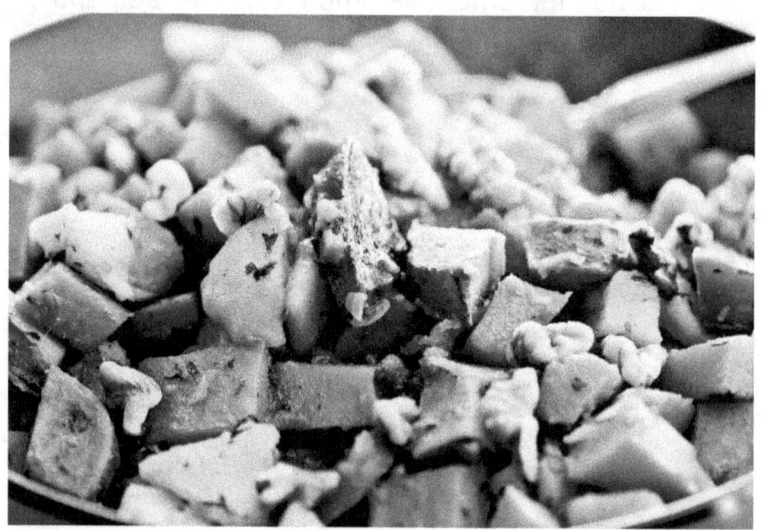

Ingredients:

1 tablespoon olive oil

1 medium yellow onion, chopped

1 cup diced cauliflower florets

½ cup diced carrot

2 medium sweet potatoes, peeled and diced

Salt and pepper to taste

¼ cup chopped walnuts

2 teaspoons chili powder

1 teaspoon dried parsley

Instructions:

1. Heat the oil in a large skillet over medium heat.
2. Add the onions, cauliflower, carrots and sweet potato – season with salt and pepper to taste.
3. Sauté the vegetables for about 5 minutes then add a few tablespoons of water to the skillet.
4. Cover the skillet and steam the vegetables for 3 to 4 minutes until just tender.
5. Stir in the walnuts, chili powder and parsley then spread the mixture evenly in the skillet.
6. Reduce heat to low and cook for 5 to 6 minutes without stirring until browned on the bottom.
7. Stir then cook for another 2 to 3 minutes and serve hot.

Almond Flour Blueberry Muffins

Servings: 12

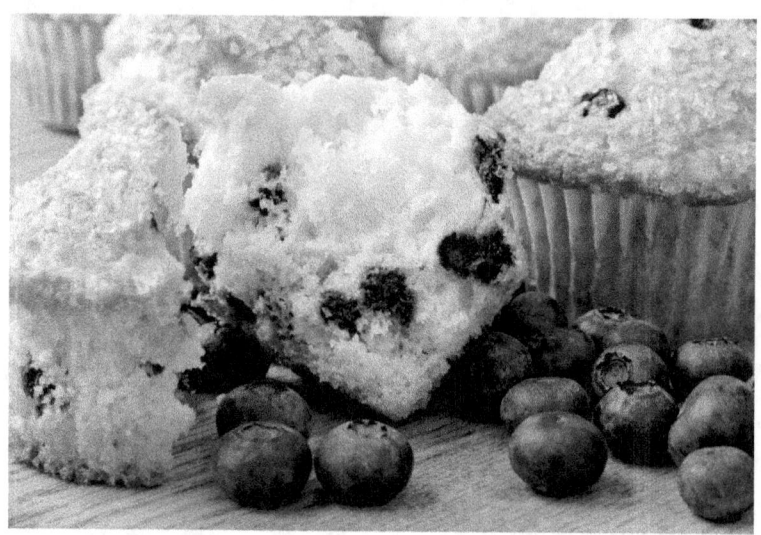

Ingredients:

2 cups almond flour

½ teaspoon baking soda

¼ teaspoon salt

2 large eggs, beaten

1 cup unsweetened applesauce

¼ cup coconut oil, melted

¼ cup maple syrup

1 ½ cups fresh blueberries

Instructions:

1. Preheat the oven to 350°F (180°C) and line a muffin pan with paper liners.
2. Combine the almond flour, baking soda and salt in a mixing bowl.
3. In a separate bowl, whisk together the eggs, applesauce, coconut oil, and maple syrup.
4. Whisk the dry ingredient into the wet until well combined then fold in the blueberries.
5. Spoon the batter into the pan, filling the cups about ¾ full.
6. Bake for 20 to 25 minutes until a knife inserted in the center comes out clean.
7. Cool the muffins for 5 minutes in the pan then turn out onto a wire rack to cool completely.

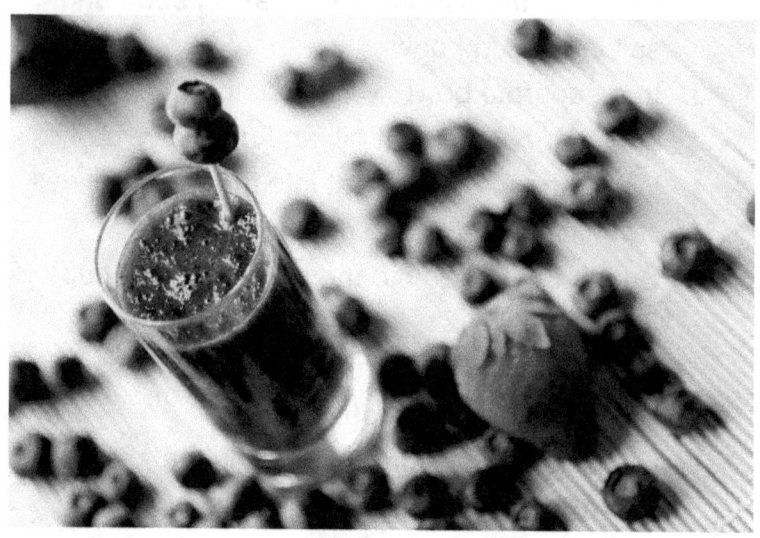

Triple Berry Coconut Smoothie

Servings: 1 to 2

Ingredients:

1 ½ cups frozen sliced strawberries

1 cup frozen blueberries

½ cup frozen raspberries or blackberries

1 medium frozen banana, peeled and sliced

1 cup unsweetened almond milk

½ cup ice cubes

2 teaspoons raw honey

Instructions:

1. Combine all of the ingredients in a high-speed blender.
2. Blend for 30 to 60 seconds until smooth and well combined.
3. Divide the smoothie amongst the two glasses and serve immediately.

Cinnamon Spiced Pumpkin Pancakes

Servings: 4

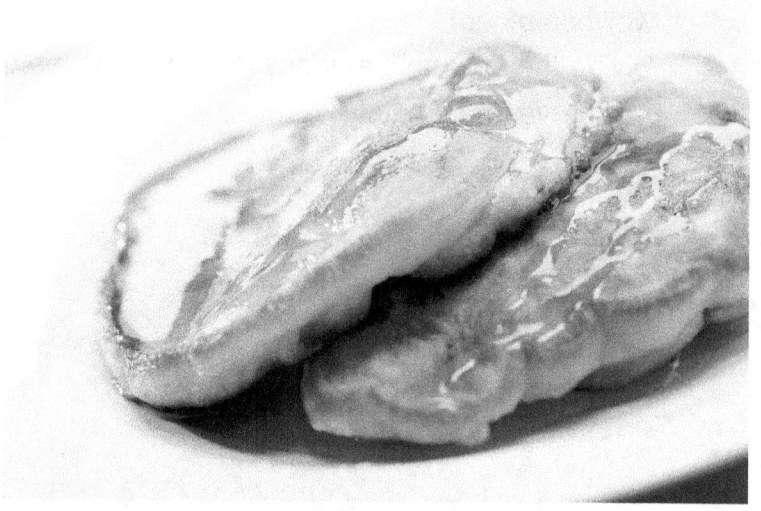

Ingredients:

1 cup pumpkin puree

6 large eggs, whisked

¼ cup plus 1 tablespoon coconut flour

1 teaspoon ground cinnamon

½ teaspoon ground nutmeg

Pinch salt

Instructions:

1. Combine the pumpkin, coconut flour, eggs, cinnamon, nutmeg and salt in a food processor.

2. Blend until smooth and well combined.
3. Heat a skillet over medium-high heat and grease with cooking oil.
4. Spoon the batter into the pan, using about 2 to 3 tablespoons per pancake.
5. Cook for 1 to 2 minutes until the underside is lightly browned.
6. Flip the pancakes and cook for another 2 minutes or until browned on the underside.
7. Transfer the pancakes to a plate to keep warm and repeat with the remaining batter.

Raspberry Coconut Muffins

Servings: 12

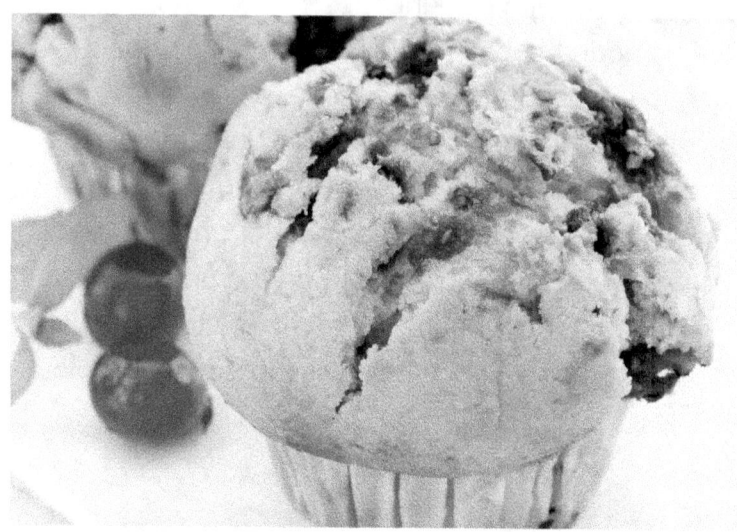

Ingredients:

2 cups almond flour

½ teaspoon baking soda

¼ teaspoon salt

2 large eggs, beaten

1 cup unsweetened applesauce

¼ cup coconut oil, melted

¼ cup maple syrup

1 cup fresh raspberries

½ cup unsweetened shredded coconut

Instructions:

1. Preheat the oven to 350°F (180°C) and line a muffin pan with paper liners.
2. Combine the almond flour, baking soda and salt in a mixing bowl.
3. In a separate bowl, whisk together the eggs, applesauce, coconut oil, and maple syrup.
4. Whisk the dry ingredient into the wet until well combined then fold in the raspberries and coconut.
5. Spoon the batter into the pan, filling the cups about ¾ full.
6. Bake for 20 to 25 minutes until a knife inserted in the center comes out clean.
7. Cool the muffins for 5 minutes in the pan then turn out onto a wire rack to cool completely.

Cream of Broccoli Soup

Servings: 4 to 6

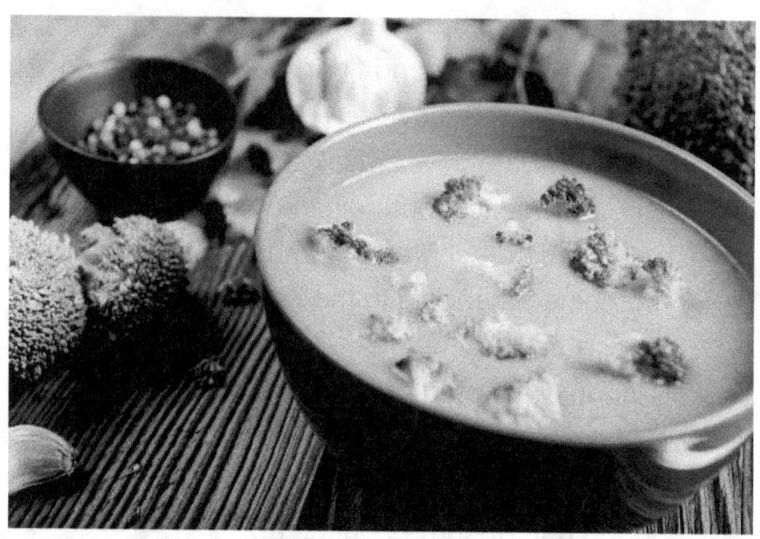

Ingredients:

1 tablespoon olive oil

1 small yellow onion, chopped

2 cloves garlic, minced

8 cups chopped broccoli florets

1 quart vegetable or chicken broth

1 cup full-fat coconut milk

Salt and pepper to taste

Instructions:

1. Heat the oil in a large saucepan over medium-high heat.
2. Add the onion, garlic and broccoli and cook for 6 to 8 minutes until tender.
3. Stir in the remaining ingredients and bring to boil.
4. Reduce heat and simmer for 22 to 25 minutes until the vegetables are tender.
5. Remove from heat then puree the soup using an immersion blender until smooth.
6. Season with salt and pepper to taste – serve hot.

Spinach Salad with Strawberries

Servings: 4

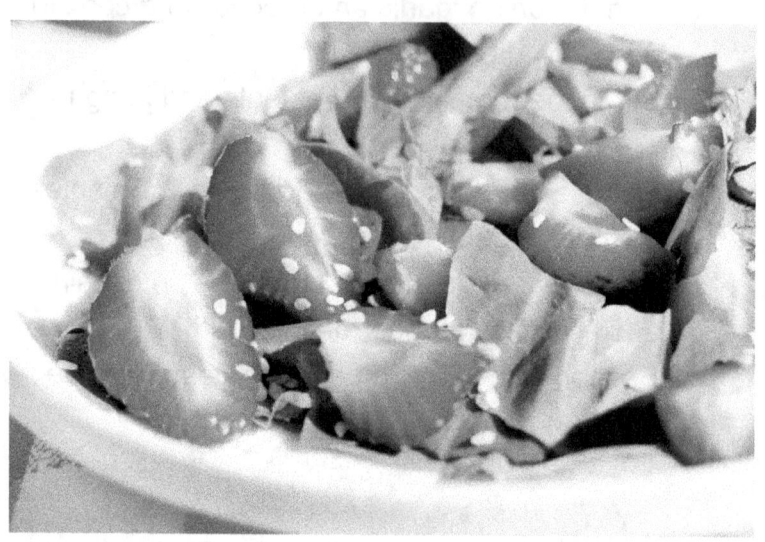

Ingredients:

6 cups fresh chopped spinach, packed

1 ¼ cups fresh diced strawberries

¼ cup extra-virgin olive oil

2 ½ tablespoons balsamic vinegar

1 tablespoon minced yellow onion

¼ teaspoon dry mustard powder

Instructions:

1. Divide the spinach among four salad plates and top with diced strawberries.

2. Combine the remaining ingredients in a small bowl.
3. Whisk until well combined then drizzle over the salads to serve.

Dairy-Free Chicken Pecan Salad

Servings: 6

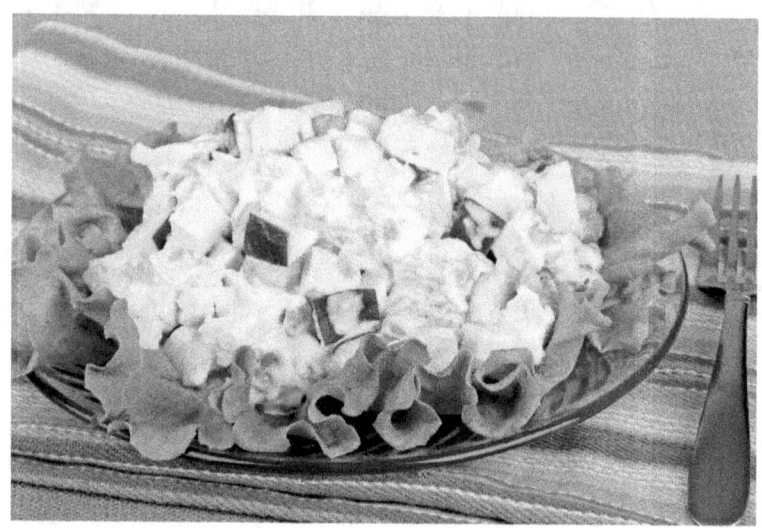

Ingredients:

1 medium ripe avocado, pitted and chopped

½ cup canned coconut milk

1 ¼ lbs. boneless skinless chicken breast, cooked and chopped

2 small red apples, cored and chopped

1 cup red seedless grapes, halved

½ cup chopped pecans

2 tablespoons fresh lemon juice

Salt and pepper to taste

Instructions:

1. Place the avocado in a mixing bowl and mash with a fork – stir in the coconut milk and whisk smooth.
2. Add the chicken, apples, grapes and pecans – toss to coat.
3. Stir in the lemon juice and season with salt and pepper to taste.
4. Chill until ready to serve – serve over a bed of lettuce.

Creamy Carrot Ginger Soup

Servings: 4 to 6

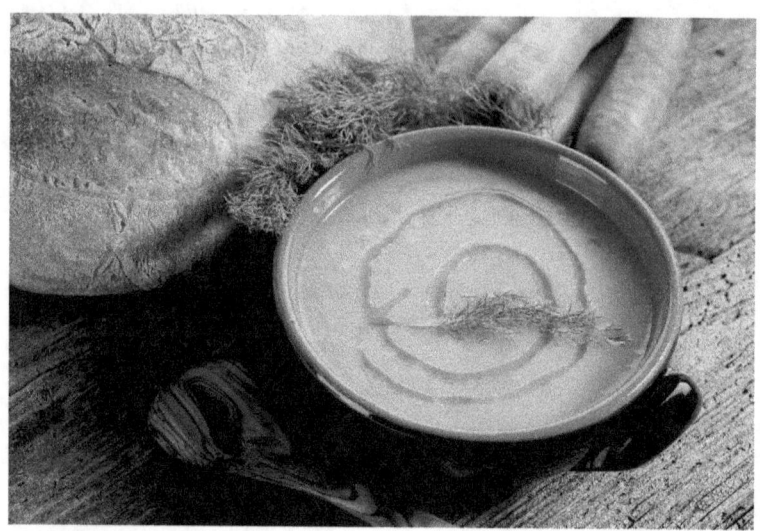

Ingredients:

1 tablespoon olive oil

1 medium yellow onion, chopped

½ tablespoon fresh grated ginger

1 lbs. fresh chopped carrots

1 medium Yukon gold potato, peeled and diced

1 quart vegetable or chicken broth

1 tablespoon fresh lemon juice

Salt and pepper to taste

Instructions:

1. Heat the oil in a large saucepan over medium-high heat.
2. Add the onion, ginger, carrots and potato then cook for 6 to 8 minutes until tender.
3. Stir in the remaining ingredients and bring to boil.
4. Reduce heat and simmer for 22 to 25 minutes until the vegetables are tender.
5. Remove from heat then puree the soup using an immersion blender until smooth.
6. Season with salt and pepper to taste – serve hot.

Spring Salad with Mango, Avocado and Walnuts

Servings: 4

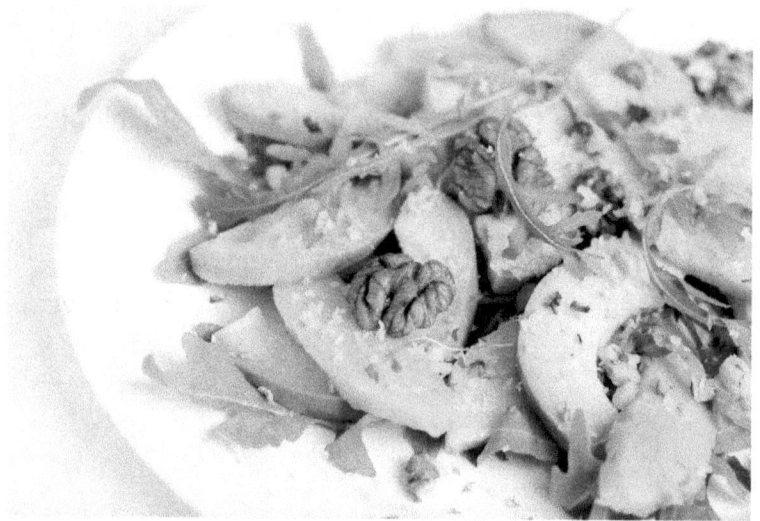

Ingredients:

6 cups fresh spring greens, packed

1 medium ripe avocado, pitted and sliced thin

1 medium mango, pitted and sliced thin

1/3 cup chopped walnuts

¼ cup extra-virgin olive oil

2 tablespoons red wine vinegar

½ tablespoon balsamic vinegar

Salt and pepper to taste

Pinch dry mustard powder

Instructions:

1. Divide the spring greens among four salad plates and top with slices of avocado and mango.
2. Sprinkle the walnuts over the salads.
3. Combine the remaining ingredients in a small bowl.
4. Whisk until well combined then drizzle over the salads to serve.

Egg Salad with Fresh Chives

Servings: 6

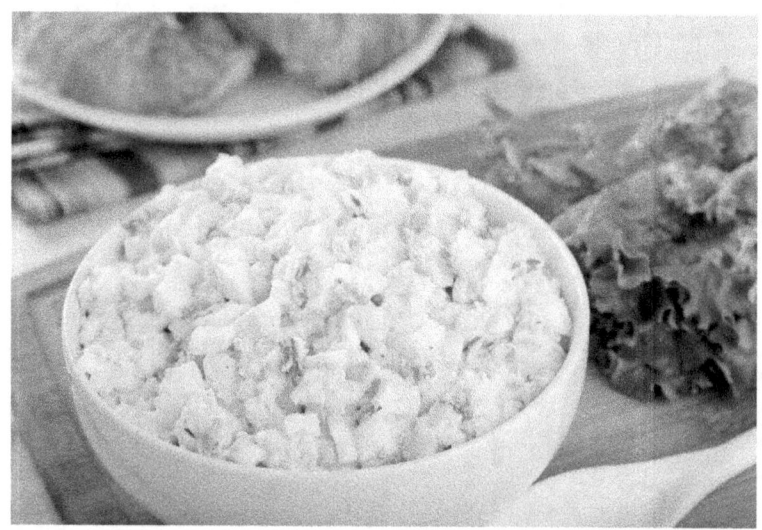

Ingredients:

10 hardboiled eggs, peeled and diced

2 large stalks celery, diced fine

¼ cup diced red onion

2 tablespoons fresh chopped chives

1 ripe avocado, pitted and mashed

2 tablespoons Dijon mustard

Salt and pepper to taste

Instructions:

1. Place the avocado in a bowl and mash with a fork – fold in the chopped eggs.
2. Stir in the remaining ingredients until well combined.
3. Chill until ready to serve.

Coconut-Crusted Baked Haddock

Servings: 6

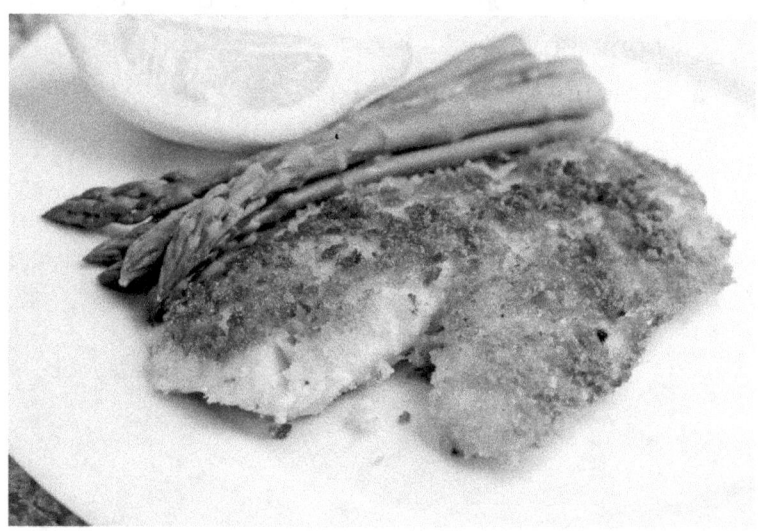

Ingredients:

6 (6-ounce) haddock fillets

1 to 2 tablespoons olive oil

Salt and pepper to taste

½ cup almond flour

½ cup unsweetened shredded coconut

1 teaspoon chili powder

Lemon wedges

Instructions:

1. Preheat the oven to 350°F (180°C)

2. Brush the fillets with olive oil and season with salt and pepper to taste.
3. Combine the almond flour, coconut and chili powder in a bowl.
4. Dredge the fillets in the coconut mixture and place them on a roasting pan.
5. Bake for 10 to 12 minutes until the flesh flakes easily with a fork.
6. Serve the fillets hot with lemon wedges.

Rosemary Roasted Chicken

Servings: 6

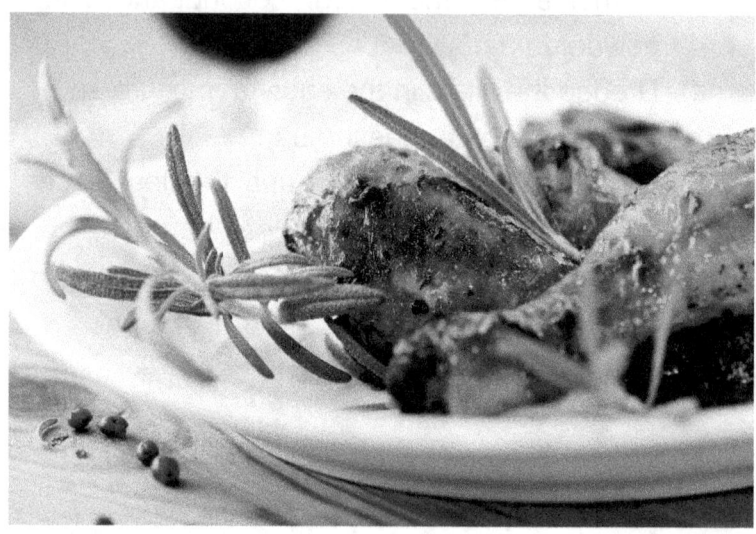

Ingredients:

2 tablespoons olive oil

2 lbs. chicken thighs and drumsticks, bone-in

Salt and pepper to taste

2 medium yellow onions, quartered

2 tablespoons fresh chopped rosemary

¼ cup chicken broth

Instructions:

1. Preheat the oven to 400°F (205°C).
2. Heat the oil in a large skillet over medium-high heat.

3. Season the chicken with salt and pepper to taste and add it to the skillet.
4. Cook for 2 to 3 minutes on each side until lightly browned.
5. Spread the onions in the bottom of a glass baking dish and arrange the chicken on top.
6. Sprinkle with rosemary and season with salt and pepper to taste.
7. Drizzle the chicken with chicken broth and roast for 30 minutes.
8. Turn the chicken and cook for another 25 to 30 minutes until cooked through.

Herb-Roasted Pork Tenderloin

Servings: 6

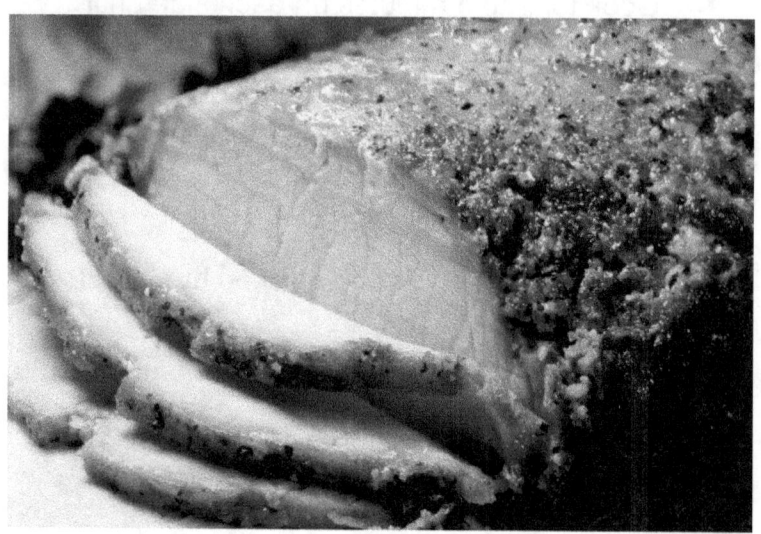

Ingredients:

2 tablespoons olive oil

3 lbs. boneless pork tenderloin

Salt and pepper to taste

1 ½ tablespoons fresh chopped rosemary

2 teaspoons dried oregano

½ teaspoon dried thyme

Instructions:

1. Preheat the oven to 400°F (205°C).
2. Heat the oil in a large skillet over medium-high heat.

3. Season the pork with salt and pepper to taste and add it to the skillet.
4. Cook for 2 to 3 minutes on each side until lightly browned.
5. Place the pork on a roasting pan skin-side down and spread the onions around it.
6. Sprinkle the herbs over the pork and roast for 30 minutes.
7. Turn the pork fat-side up and roast for another 22 to 25 minutes until it registers an internal temperature of 155°F.
8. Transfer the pork to a cutting board and let rest for 10 minutes before slicing.

Bacon-Wrapped Scallops

Servings: 4 to 6

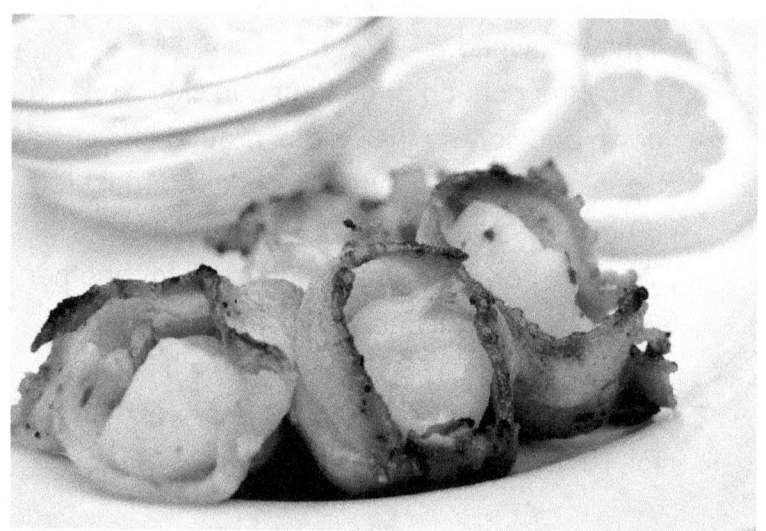

Ingredients:

1 ½ lbs. large scallops, uncooked

½ lbs. thinly sliced bacon

Chili powder to taste

Salt and pepper to taste

Instructions:

1. Preheat the broiler in your oven to high heat.
2. Wrap the scallops in slices of bacon and use wooden toothpicks to secure them.
3. Arrange the scallops on a roasting pan and sprinkle with chili powder.

4. Season with salt and pepper to taste and broil for 10 to 15 minutes until the scallops are cooked through and the bacon is crisp.

Easy Homemade Meatloaf

Servings: 6

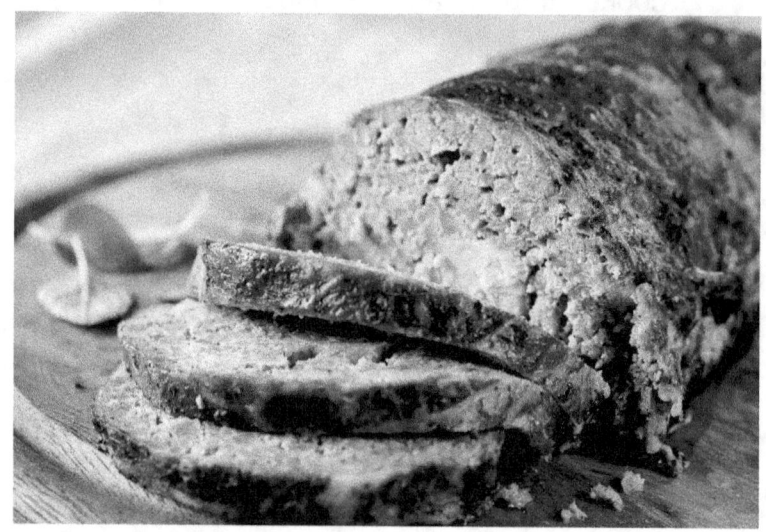

Ingredients:

1 lbs. lean ground beef

½ lbs. ground lamb or pork

2/3 cup almond flour

2 large eggs

1/3 cup tomato sauce

1 ½ tablespoons Dijon mustard

2 teaspoons dried Italian seasoning

Salt and pepper to taste

Instructions:

1. Preheat the oven to 400°F (205°C) and lightly grease a loaf pan with cooking spray.
2. Combine all of the ingredients in a mixing bowl and stir well.
3. Press the mixture into the loaf pan as evenly as possible.
4. Bake for 45 to 55 minutes until the internal temperature registers 165°F.
5. Let the meatloaf rest for 10 minutes then turn out and slice to serve.

Spicy Chipotle Turkey Burgers

Servings: 4

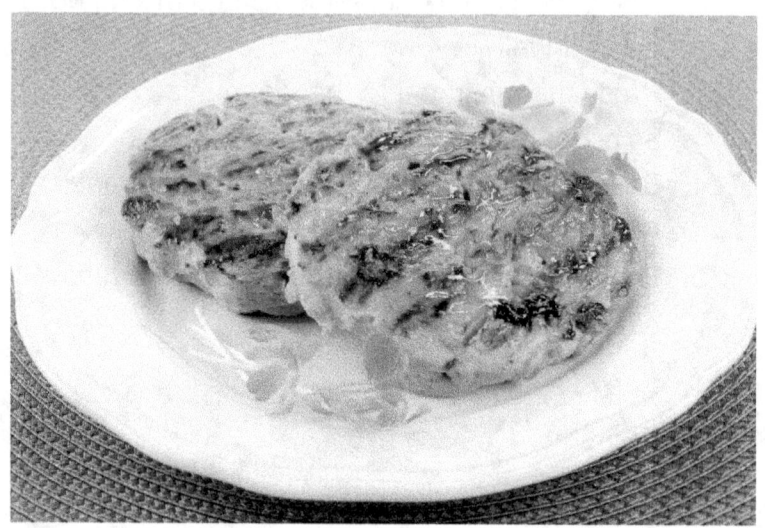

Ingredients:

1 lbs. lean ground turkey

½ cup diced yellow onion

¼ cup almond flour

1 large egg, whisked

1 tablespoon chilies in chipotle sauce, chopped

1 teaspoon chipotle chili powder

Salt and pepper to taste

Instructions:

1. Preheat the broiler to high heat.

2. Combine the ingredients in a mixing bowl and stir until well combined.
3. Divide the mixture into four even-sized patties and place them on a broiler pan.
4. Broil for 4 to 5 minutes on each side until cooked through.
5. Serve the patties hot on paleo-friendly sandwich buns.

Cinnamon Baked Bananas

Servings: 5 to 6

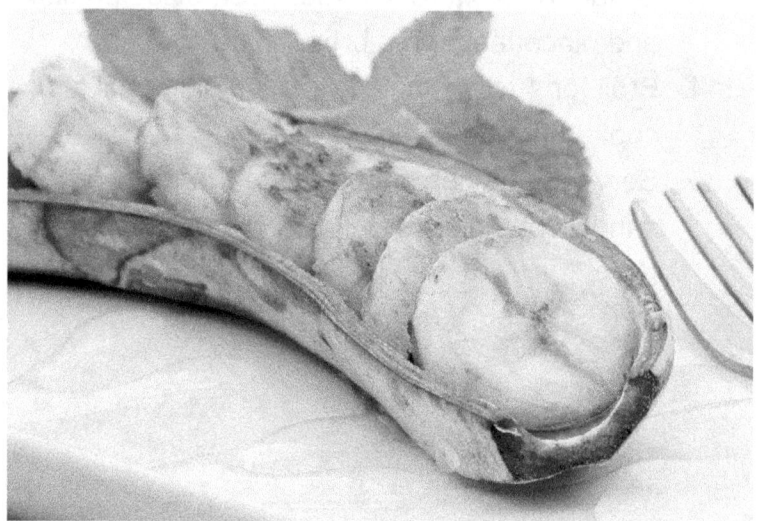

Ingredients:

6 medium ripe bananas, peeled and sliced

3 tablespoons raw honey

1 teaspoon ground cinnamon

Instructions:

1. Preheat the oven to 350°F (180°C) and grease a square glass baking dish.
2. Toss the bananas with the honey and cinnamon.
3. Spread the bananas in the baking dish and bake for 15 to 20 minutes until tender.

Chocolate Fudge Brownies

Servings: 12 to 16

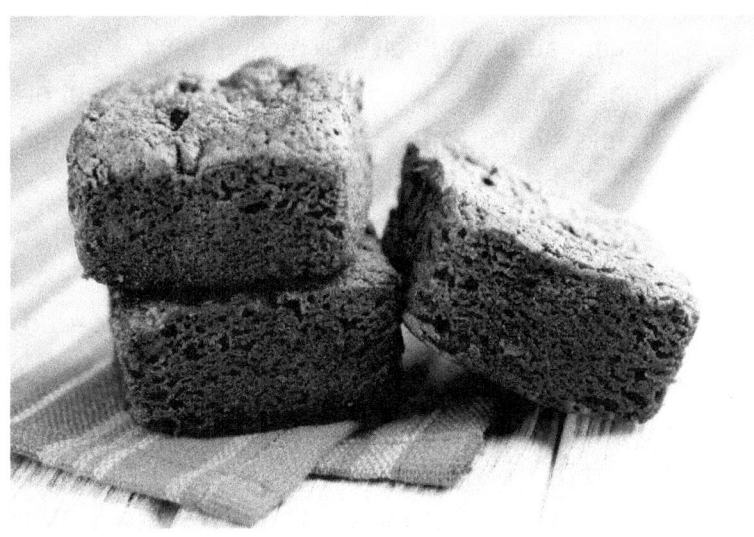

Ingredients:

½ cup sifted coconut flour

½ cup unsweetened cocoa powder

½ teaspoon baking soda

¼ teaspoon salt

½ cup plus 2 tablespoons coconut oil, melted

½ cup maple syrup

3 large eggs, beaten

½ tablespoon vanilla extract

Instructions:

1. Preheat the oven to 300°F (150°C) and grease an 8x8-inch glass baking dish.
2. Combine the coconut flour, cocoa powder, baking soda and salt in a mixing bowl.
3. In another bowl, whisk together the coconut oil, maple syrup, eggs and vanilla extract until well combined.
4. Stir in the dry ingredients until smooth then spread in the baking dish.
5. Bake for 30 to 35 minutes until a knife inserted in the center comes out clean.
6. Cool the brownies completely before cutting into squares.

Coconut Vanilla Cupcakes

Servings: 12

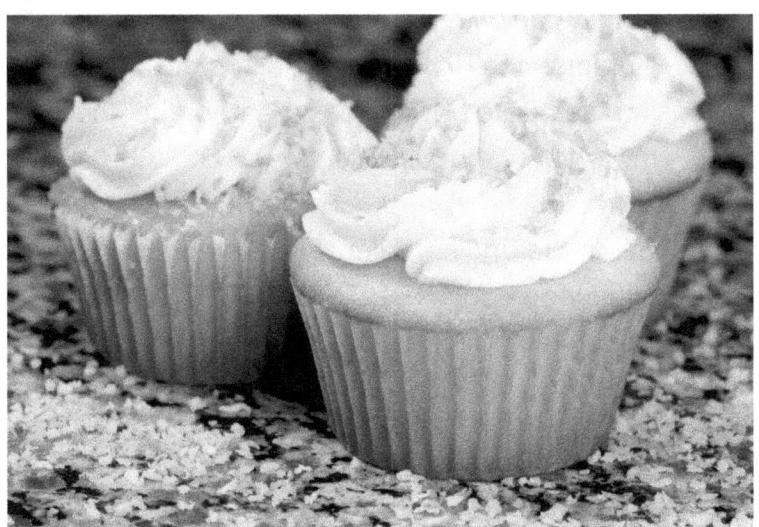

Ingredients:

¾ cups almond flour

2/3 cup sifted coconut flour

1 teaspoon baking soda

½ teaspoon salt

2/3 cup canned coconut milk

½ cup raw honey

2 tablespoons coconut oil

6 large eggs, beaten

2 teaspoons vanilla extract

Instructions:

1. Preheat the oven to 350°F (180°C) and line a muffin pan with paper liners.
2. Combine the dry ingredients in a mixing bowl.
3. In a separate bowl, whisk together the coconut milk, honey, coconut oil, honey and vanilla extract.
4. Stir in the dry ingredients until smooth and well combined – fold in the coconut.
5. Spoon the mixture into the muffin pan, filling the cups 2/3 full.
6. Bake for 20 to 25 minutes until a knife inserted in the center comes out clean.
7. Cool for 5 minutes in the pan then turn out onto a wire rack to cool completely.

Blueberry Almond Flour Crisp

Servings: 4 to 6

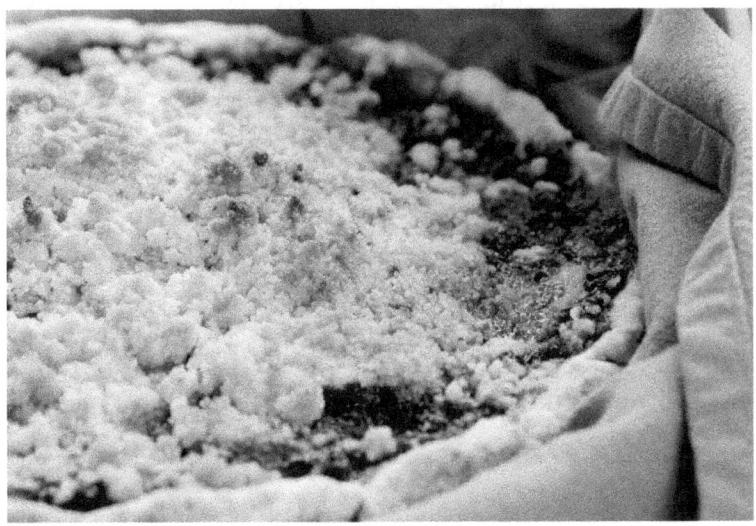

Ingredients:

6 cups fresh blueberries

1 tablespoon arrowroot powder

1 cup almond flour

½ cup almond, finely chopped

1/3 cup coconut oil

½ teaspoon ground cinnamon

Instructions:

1. Preheat the oven to 375°F (190°C) and grease a glass pie plate.

2. Toss the blueberries with arrowroot powder and spread in the pie plate.
3. Combine the remaining ingredients in a mixing bowl to form a crumbled mixture.
4. Sprinkle the mixture over the berries and bake for 20 minutes until hot and bubbling.

Avocado Chocolate Mousse

Servings: 6

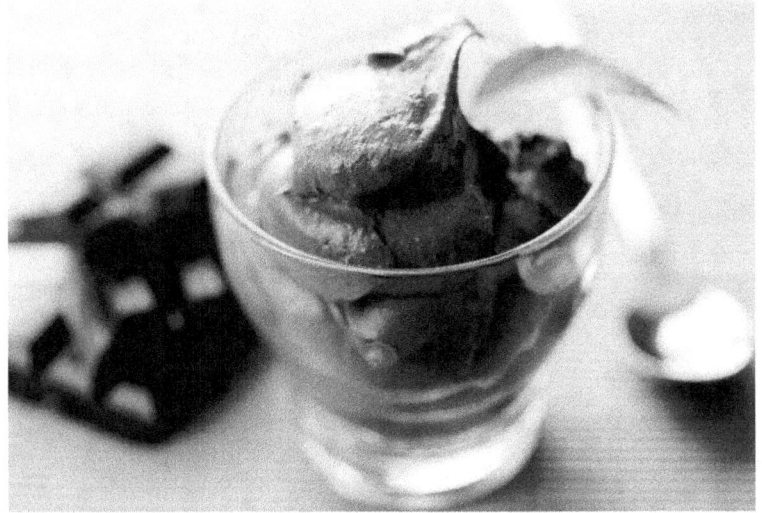

Ingredients:

3 medium ripe avocados, pitted and chopped

½ cup canned coconut milk

1/3 cup raw honey

1/3 cup unsweetened cocoa powder

1 teaspoon vanilla extract

Instructions:

1. Combine the avocado, coconut milk, honey, cocoa powder and vanilla in a food processor.
2. Blend until smooth and well combined.

3. Spoon the mixture into dessert cups and chill until ready to serve.

Conclusion

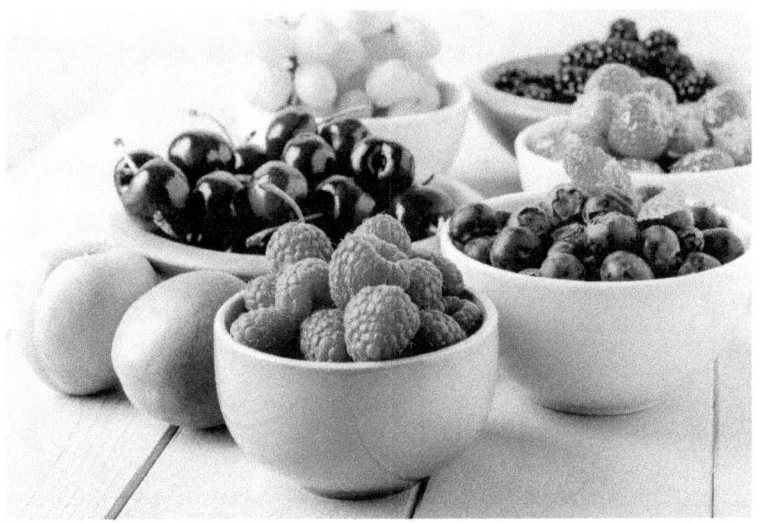

After reading this book, you should have a basic understanding of the Paleo Diet including a list of foods to eat and avoid. The Paleo Diet is an excellent tool for weight loss and many people use it as a treatment for chronic diseases. If you are ready to give the Paleo Diet a try this book is the perfect place to start. In addition to receive a quick-start guide to the Paleo Diet you have also received a collection of delicious Paleo recipes. To get started with the Paleo Diet simply pick a recipe from this book and give it a try. You won't be disappointed.